Almost All Carb
"Diet"

Carb-Advantageous and Carb-A-Licious
Ideas, Attitudes and the FREEDOM
to Enjoy Paradise, Inside and Out

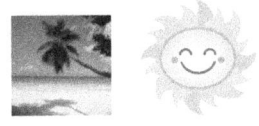

Maryann Fenicato, Esq., Ph.D.

DEDICATION

This book is dedicated to anyone who wants to ENJOY life,
FEEL great and FREE,
because this is not a "diet," but a way of life, a 'way to be!

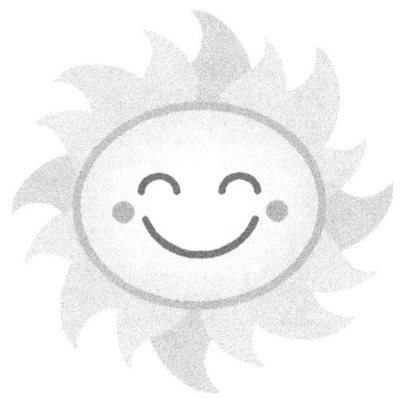

CONTENTS

ACKNOWLEDGMENTS

As always, sincerest gratitude to my best friends, Bobbie, Dave and Nancy. Special thanks Ginger and all her wonderful friends, Sue, and anyone who helps me in the slightest way, which can mean so much, here's hoping you get it back from God or Karma 10-fold.

Specific appreciation to all the wonderful people who complimentarily call me "the runner," especially those who understand that my morning run is much more than mere exercise. I was "born to run," literally, so it's so nice to be known and appreciated for something that I really enjoy so much.

May you enjoy the same.

1
INTRODUCTION

For some of us, carbs are like chocolate. Yeah!

But, with all due respect to chocolate bliss, unlike it, they do not provide regrettable temporary pleasure that would have to be lived down or hard to eliminate later. No, they BURN OFF very easy and make you feel great AFTERWARD. How cool is that!

They pep you up BEFORE you even eat them, because as you look forward to them EXCITEDLY, your correct attitude powers them up and makes them buzz with electric energy. So, you see there is more to this than meets the eye. Approaching just about anything with the right attitude is key.

So, this book will shed light on the right attitude to have towards related issues, both for yourself and others, so that all your efforts do not backfire, rather, provide maximum lasting benefit. Understanding deeper reasons, especially emotional ones, as to why certain ideas work for you or others is another key.

Many ideas, in fact, will be shared, by someone who cares. Words can be wings. Even if you've tried everything else, amazing healings can be done by just one.

This book does not, however, have all the answers. In saying that, I am not just being humble or honest, rather, I encourage all of you to supplement and try out other things, and do them as well. These are simply ideas that have worked well for me, and since I receive so many compliments especially on my running, I love to share and help others find paradise, inside and out.

But, please understand that the main goal if this book is not to suggest temporary ideas, no matter how good, rather, a pervasive attitude and a much better, lasting way of life. If a person only treats symptoms, not the real cause of a problem, or puts a bucket under a leaky roof without fixing the actual roof, it will fail. So, this book will guide you to go deeper inside your heart, mind and soul, to find out what it is that is really holding back your health. As a wise lady once said to me, "It's not WHAT ails you, but WHO." She meant that stress, especially when triggered by other people whom you can never please, get away from, etc., is often the true underlying problem, the emotional escalator. So, a person may NEVER find a "diet" that works until you realize the true cause and start doing something about that!

Yet, this book will also shine a spiritual light that may surprise you. For instance, did it ever occur to you that the "Lord's Prayer," which asks God to "give us our daily BREAD," might be expressly, specifically requesting carbs! How about that? To feed Moses's starving gang as they journeyed to their Promised Land, God provided "manna," that is, BREAD, from heaven. Another clue?

Heaven is, in fact, this book's biggest goal—to show you how to create it for yourself, right here on earth. It also explains how to obtain lasting inner peace, as well as the ultimate Peace of Christ.

Yet, some will only find it if they finally step up to making the huge lifestyle changes that they have always wanted, dreamed of, or unfortunately, forcefully repressed, especially by listening to others who may NOT have your best interests in mind. They may have ulterior motives to keep you from the right diet or life you deserve, undermining not just your diet, but your whole life and health.

So, this book will also help you see that "WHO" ails you might just be YOU, yourself.

Who—You?

Who knew?

If so, no worries, because the golden key to that will be handed to you, too. So, read on, rise to a higher attitude, a better you, keeping yourself focused on God, and true FREEDOM!

Bottom line: Be Free!

2
CARB-VANTAGEOUS!

A. The Right Carbs

Let's leave long, boring, waste-of-time discussions of "good versus bad" carbs alone. Why even "go there" when "carb-vantageous" quickly and easily fit two cool categories: 1) comfort and 2) crunch.

1. Comfort

"Comfort" carbs fit a bigger "comfort foods" category we know so well, which include lots of other things that hold or keep you from feeling hungry for quite a while, and of course, make a person feel mighty fine and "warm and fuzzy" inside. The key, however, is to pick those that don't have lots of difficult-to-burn off calories.

For instance, macaroni and cheese can certainly be a yummy treat, keeping hunger at bay and your tummy very happy, but the cheese sauce may contain too many calories. So instead of eating plain mac, why not simply go for stuff that ALREADY tastes great on its own without many, if any, embellishments, especially **soft breads, big soft pretzels, and of course, bagels**. Sweet sigh!

Nor would there be any need to settle for plain stuff, because those with few additions, such as sesame or poppy seeds, can be really tasty, without compromising calories. Many taste so good on their own without any enhancements that the old adage of "less is more" would really be incredibly correct.

Best of all, while this book will use the word, "comfort" to mainly mean soft bread and bagels avoiding problematic additions, feel free to experiment, find what works for you, and add them into this flexible category. In fact, each person should have the power and control, yet enjoy the fun, of tailoring it to perfectly fit themselves.

Enjoy that freedom!

2. Crunch

Crunchy carbs come in lots of varieties, as well, but we will focus on those that make great snacks—putting pep in your step with each pop, not disadvantageous calories. For instance, **certain cereals like corn flakes, rice krispies, corn pops, and of course, mini hard pretzels**, taste great on their own without extra calories of add-ins, while providing a literal snap, crackle and pop. Yet, again, certain embellishments, such as spices containing hardly any calories, etc. can make quite a difference.

Instead of comfort, these give us something just as great, on a different level, a priceless feeling of freedom, because they have even fewer calories, so one can eat MORE of them. So, they provide an outlet for the psychological need for "more" that we all have, as long as we do not take it too far.

Feel free!

What a feeling!

Once again, have fun experimenting to find the right ones for you. Create or carve out a more specific or expansive personal category.

3. The Key to Both Categories

The most important aspect of both categories is, however, how you feel AFTERWARD. Sure, many foods make you feel awesome while you're eating them, but what happens later? You should still feel great, if not very good, hours later. If not, and especially if you feel tired, sleepy, irritable, etc., immediately afterwards, you need to go back and make better choices.

4. Because You're Worth It!

Please realize that a lot of "trial and error" during experimentation is not only quite normal, but very much expected, until you find the perfect fit. So, know ahead of time that even the best choices may not turn out well, and certain results may not be obvious or any fault of your own. You'll never really know until you try, and even if it takes a while, the results will be "worth it," because YOU are.

B. All the Right Moves

Now that we know the right carbs to pick, to make them optimum, we must discuss when, where, why and how to eat them.

1. No Unwanted Fillers!

Most people think of eating bread as an unwanted addition to on otherwise wonderful meal, something they have to do, not something they want to, or prefer over the rest. If done that way, with the wrong attitude, they can certainly seem to fill you up "too much," and be detrimental in many ways.

2. Bread is Basic

Instead, bread should be seen as basic, the base, keystone or main part of one or more meals, when the comfort stuff would be key.

In fact, especially for those of us that love and look forward to them more than anything else, feel free to have one meal that is mostly carbs, one that is half, and a third when carbs are an add-on.

Here are more reasons why, going lower and way high:

First, let's take a better look at what has come to be considered a lowly or negative expression, "bread and water." Yes, honestly and humbly, that concerns prison rations, but WHY would bread even be chosen for something like that in the first place? The answers are advantageous for both sides, survival, reasonable cost, etc.

3. Give Us Our Daily Bread

Next, notice that as taught to us by Jesus, Himself, "Lord's Prayer" specifically asks God to "give us our daily BREAD." Humn...! He may very well have meant that literally, and practically, for common sense, as well as a highly spiritual, request!

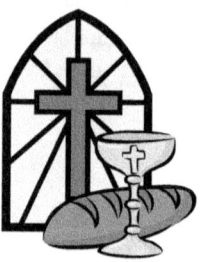

<u>Jovial, spiritual note</u>: Later the same day that I drafted this section, an acquaintance I never thought I'd ever hear from again suddenly emailed, providing the specific Bible citation for that prayer: Matthew 6:11. Tell me that was a coincidence! Besides mere serendipity, it may have been a sign or a gift from God, a "God-incidence." That made me feel great, too, as if in addition to the quote, I received His approval, a sign that He's behind and backing all this. When God's "got your back," it can be better than carbs!

4. Beyond Bread Alone

Yet, since even Jesus said, "Man does not live on bread alone," (Matthew 4:4, Luke 4:4 and Deuteronomy 8:3) at least one or two of your three main meals should certainly focus on the other food groups--what else to eat and include will be totally up to each of you. Yet, other carbs should be added as wonderful light energy snacks for continued benefits throughout the day.

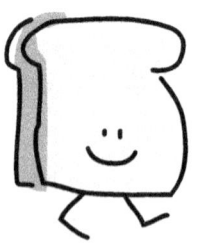

5. Snappy Snacks

To keep yourself carb-happy and snappy, that is, full of easily burned-off energy, also enjoy one or two crunchy snacks per day. In so doing, you will be spreading the wealth out incrementally, giving yourself a boost when you need and can best use it, as well as when you can most easily ease off the calories.

Jovial note: Many people think or worry too much, so these snacks are just perfect, easily eliminated by that kind of "mental" activity. And such a spread-out schedule form-fits those who never stop!

Seriously, though, these ideas are just the ticket for "office types," who need to keep their energy up throughout their work day, which can go beyond 9-5, yet fit their mostly sedentary work, which could not burn off massive calories easily or effectively. Notice that even running a "marathon" during lunch would not work, making them most likely too tired to finish the day, etc.

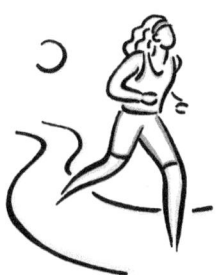

So, now that we'd discussed which carbs and the best ways to enjoy them that would be optimum and most advantageous, next, let's do basically the same with exercise.

Maryann Fenicato, Esq., Ph.D.

3
LET'S GET PHYSICAL!

A. First, Let's Laugh

As I was about to choose the title for this section, I could hear the lyrics of that 80's exercise anthem playing in my head. No, I was NOT fond of it, let alone Richard Simmons' television antics, or Jane Fonda's video workouts, etc. Better to leave it alone, right?

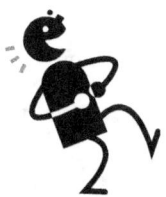

B. Now, Let's Learn

But, then it suddenly occurred to me that it's still the perfect title for this section, for a different reason--it quickly conveys the idea that we can look back and laugh, and chose better things now. Remembering makes better options available now even sweeter.

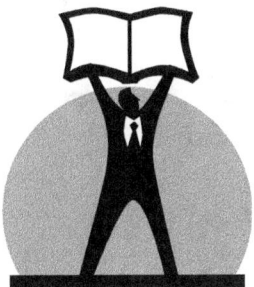

C. Successful Strategies

1. No Long. Difficult Workouts!

One of the biggest mistakes people certainly did back then and still do now, is opt for long, difficult workouts. Thinking "no pain, no gain," was the answer, it is actually wrong to do too much all at once, to get it out of the way. If it tires you out physically as well as emotionally, it can ruin the rest of your day, and the things you chose to do as a result, can undermine all your burdensome efforts.

A much better idea is to do things in the morning, that rev or pep you up enough to get you rolling or your motor running. That way, you can and will still want to do more things throughout your day, spreading it out for maximum benefit. For instance, instead of running a long marathon in the morning, even if you would and could, it would be more advisable to do a shorter run then, and other things later on in shorter amounts, such as a walk mid-day and perhaps another in the evening.

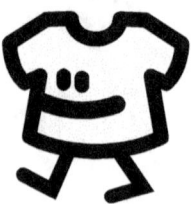

Now, it is certainly true that some people only have a certain limited amount of time to exercise, so they might want to duke it out big-time then, burning as many calories as they can. That certainly seems like a great idea, but we must realize that our physical bodies and our mental and emotional well-being go hand-in-hand. After such a physical workout, would such a person still be at their best intellectually? You get the idea—better to find a proper balance, which each person must do for themselves.

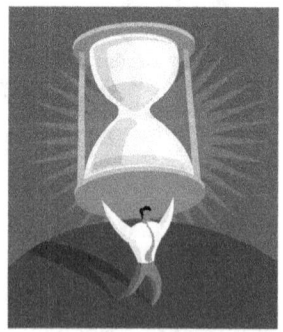

2. Small Stuff Adds Up!

Especially on days that longer workouts are not possible, skipping entire days, is not a good idea. Yes, certain pre-designated days of rest are very important, but this means more. Instead of going total cold-turkey, carve out smaller stuff, which can mean so much.

3. Outside Dependence

Another one of the biggest mistakes I see people make is to depend on exercise that must be done outside or with other people. Yes, it can definitely be more fun to run outside under blue skies and sunshine, but what about rain or other adverse weather? Doing something inside will be more beneficial than nothing.

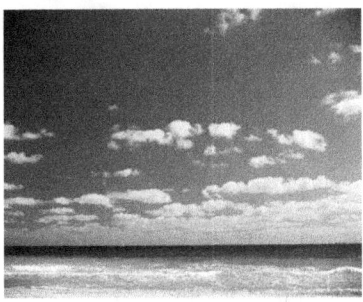

4. Social Dependence

Same for social stuff. Exercise can obviously be more fun when done with other people, but what if they cancel? Much better to do solitary stuff than be dependent on anyone else.

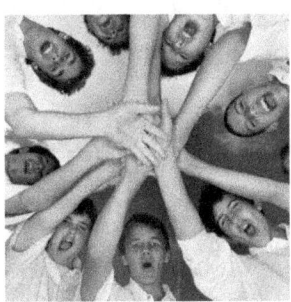

5. Gyms and "Being Seen"

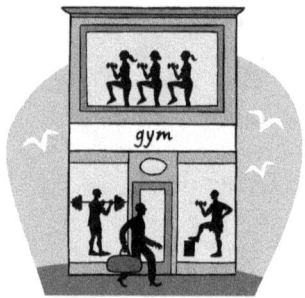

Get this: Gyms and libraries actually have common elements. Some people think they need them, and others misuse them!

<u>Jovial note</u>:   Both have advantages, which can interrelate, such as getting yourself away from noise, other people, your phone, T.V., computer or even your ... refrigerator!

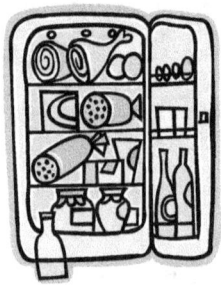

Such places can also have beneficial machines, people and other types of motivation, etc.

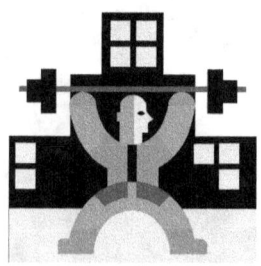

But, they can be used for the wrong reasons, especially only "being seen," without doing any work. And, that can backfire if a person is not already at their optimum weight, conditioning, etc.

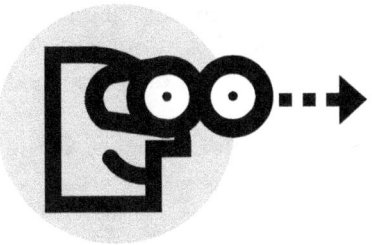

Yet, what may go unnoticed is all the time and trouble it takes to go and come back, to dress correctly, travel, etc. All of that temporal effort could be better used perhaps at home. So, before you go, ask yourself why and if you really need any of that, at all.

6.   How Others See You

No matter how long I live, one thing I may never "get over" is the jaded assumption that exercise is really done as an advertisement. I used to think that only male, dirty-old-man geezers or "peeping Toms" who get far too much of a "kick" out of modern bathing suits, were having even more of personal a "field day" with today's exercise apparel, but many women and younger people of both sexes jump to such stupid conclusions, too. Since it may not be possible to enlighten all of them, while you are exercising, you can look away from them, down at the ground, and especially very serious about, or very "into" what you're doing. That works well.

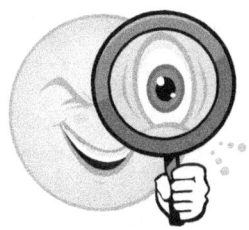

Yet, the best way to get your head around it, so that it does not deter you, is to understand that it's not really about you, but them.

I will include another paragraph about this because it can be very detrimental to people who do NOT get that treatment. Some actually want that to happen, then get upset if it does not, perhaps even giving up. Some undermine their endeavors by getting jealous of those who do. Instead, they could work inside or alone until they get to a point where they could go out and have that happen.

7. "Military" and Isometric Options

Our various military branches are pretty smart! They have figured out and require only a select few specific physical training exercises that achieve awesome results, yet can be done easily, just about any time and anywhere, and with hardly anyone or anything else.

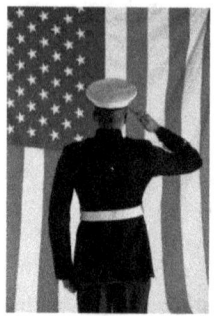 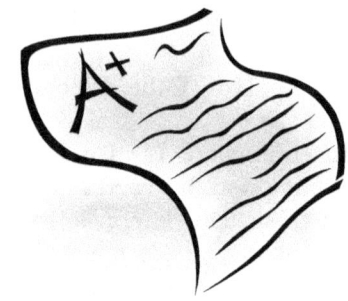

Notice that running only takes a pair of tennis shoes, sit-ups only require something to brace yourself on, if at all, and push-ups can be done almost anywhere, on just about any inside floor or outside ground. So, before you spend lots of money on any type of exercise aids or accessories, big or small, think again. They may make it more fun or worthwhile for some people, but for all, are not really necessary.

Moreover, some of those exercises, especially push-ups, are actually isometric exercises. So, before purchasing anything else, research what else could cost-effectively be accomplished with things you already have. For instance, amazing exercises or great stretches, can be done while standing within an open doorway, pushing against it. And, even if you do get other stuff, it is nice to have other options, especially when and if they suddenly stop working.

8. "Boot Camps"

<u>Jovial note</u>: Since I personally attended ARMY ROTC Basic Camp in Fort Knox, Kentucky in 1987, although I was a rare person who actually enjoyed it for many reasons, but mostly because I was treated with impressed respect (yes, I have proof), I get a kick out of watching "boot camp" training done by civilians for others. Patterned after the real stuff, it is die-hard early and arduous, so on one hand, it can get quick results. But, as discussed above, difficult workouts, especially if done at a time of day that people may not normally do or would never voluntarily choose at all, could really undermine a whole life. So, treating them as temporary stop-gaps, and finding a more moderate way of life afterward, would be wise.

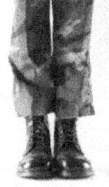 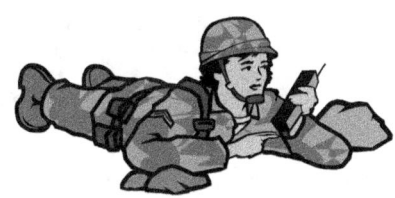

9. Other Kinds of "Copy Cats"

Before you go gung-ho about any kind of advice, diet, exercise, or otherwise, please remember that "curiosity killed the cat," and cats have nine lives, whereas you just have one! So, look at any and all advice, no matter how seemingly nice, even in this book (how about that!), with eyes wide open!

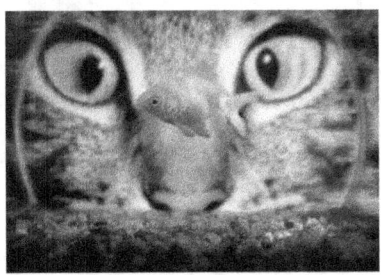

Surprised?

Don't be. Here's why:

Another huge mistake I see people make is to assume that if a person does something well, they must have some sort of magic secret, so if they could just figure it out, and go do it themselves, it would work instantaneously, like a charm. Instead, there is hardly ever just one easy answer to things like diets and exercise, so if they seem easy, they have most likely become easy, but only after long, hard or difficult periods of experimentation, etc.

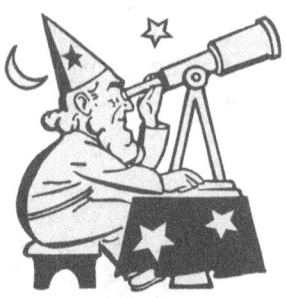

Again, the problem with adverse results can go much deeper. If a person tries something that seems to work so well for someone else, but fails miserably, they can not only give up on that particular idea, but on the exercise in general, and sometimes on themselves. So, watching others and expecting the same quick results can have a terrible impact on a person's entire self-worth or self-esteem, potentially causing them act out and/or do other regrettable things.

Parsing it for educational enlightenment, notice that trying out something new is not the problem, so please do experiment. Rather, the problem is the expectation of similar or perfect results.

Jovial note: Leading by example, and perhaps even entertaining, here's an example from my own life. After I won two "Outstanding Professor of the Year" awards from PITT, a certain college asked me to teach there, too. I caught wind from the local gossip grapevine that I had not been hired to teach the students, rather the other teachers—get me? They were out to figure out my secret and copy it themselves. And, yes, they somehow assumed there was just one. So, I taught well, and had a wonderful time, as did my students, but purposefully did it quite differently. Knowing what they were up to, I even specifically used personal examples from my life, which they, the kind of people who just try to copy others without ever accomplishing anything themselves, couldn't copy. Nor did they even know that providing personal examples is actually expected, if not required, because a good teacher goes "beyond the book," providing personal stories and examples to show students how the principles taught could be applied to their own real lives. A great one "thinks outside the box," aka the required textbook, entirely. So, although they did correctly figure out my one-word ubiquitous goal, "inspiration," they had no idea how to copy it.

Their error was trying to copy it in the first place, yet get similar results! They should have used my inspiration AS inspiration FOR THEM, to find something ELSE that works well FOR THEM.

So, here's another humble, honest surprise:

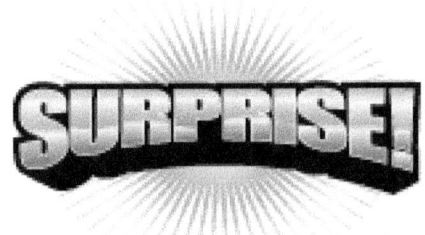

Ready?

This book does not have all the answers.

All of its ideas may not work for each of you.

They are NOT supposed to.

Instead, treat them as stars, guiding you to your promised land.

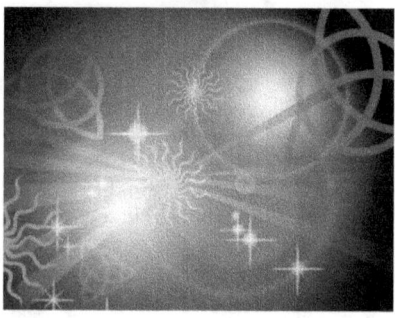

Like Moses, I can't really take you there, I can only show you the way, shining a bright light on, and sharing those that have worked well for me, but advising you that they can't be treated as quick magical fixes. Instead, you must work them out to fit each of you.

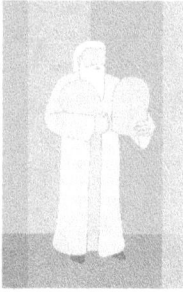

10. Myth of Ease

Another silly assumption I see all the time, especially here in Key West, is that if someone is doing something well, especially if they smile or seem happy as they do it, it must be so easy for them, like falling off a log, requiring no hard effort. Once again, the assumers undermine their own lives by getting jealous. Here's the real deal:

Certainly, some things come easier for some people, not others. Yet, hardly anything is so easy that it does not require lots of effort. Such effort may have been done long ago, so things are easy now, but that does not mean a difficult learning curve was skipped!

<u>Jovial note</u>: I used to be "dumb" enough to attend yoga classes, that is, at a studio outside with teachers and other students. I could

already do most of the poses, and even some of the more difficult ones came naturally once the teachers explained them to me. So, the teachers were right in saying that I was a "natural yogi." But, certain students wrongly assumed that I was "born yesterday," as if I had never done any of it, so it was easy as magic.

They were so jealous that even after I explained that I had done it at home, by myself, for at least 6 years (even more by now), and that I had terrible spine problems that made me want and need to experiment with the more difficult stuff, they didn't believe me. But, the truth was that some of them wanted the limelight.

I really thought one or more poses would fix my spine, if I could just find the right one, the secret I could copy—sound familiar? I was also so hurt that a "sanctuary" and all the friends I thought I'd made was not the safe haven I thought it would be So, it was difficult to I choose to be the "bigger man" and walk way.

Now, I am VERY glad I did, because if I hadn't resumed experimenting on my own at home, I never would've figured out a far more difficult twist, literally, on the most difficult pose taught to me there, which really does keep my spine in line.

Here's a picture of me doing it, touching my toe to my "third eye."

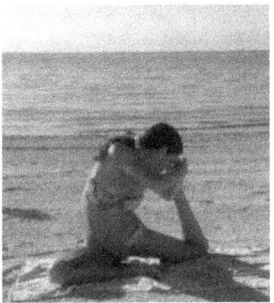

Although I always have lots of pain in other areas, at least the terrible, debilitating stabbing sciatic pain has stopped. Upon getting treatment outside of town, I've also stopped going to the chiropractors completely! How about that!

So, see this humble, jovial story as an example of how easy it is for anyone, even this humble, honest author, to attempt a quick fix. Attempting is not the problem; expecting it is. But, giving up is worst of all, so never, ever give up!

11. Driven

Another reason why it can be quite foolish to try to copy someone else yet expect similar results, or assume things come so easy for others, is they may be driven by EMOTIONAL reasons. Many people don't just do diets or exercise for the typical reasons. Yes, some do it for selfish narcissistic reasons, to be "seen" by others, etc., but others have incredible good passions. Some are driven like a moth to a flame, perhaps even to their Divine destiny.

For example, a runner might reminisce past "glory days" of winning a prize or surprisingly impressing people. Others may be taking or letting something out in a positive way, such as pretending the pavement they run on is a terrible person's face (neighbor, boss, etc.), so they enjoy pounding it with every step! But, it could also be a time or situation when they can really unburden their problems, feeling free as a bird, soaring on a runner's high, literally, in more way than one.

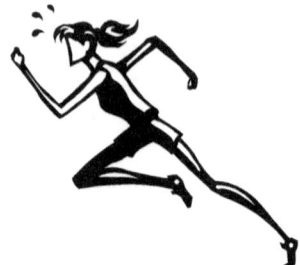 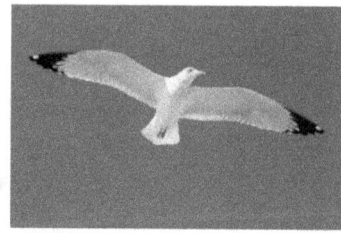

Certainly, physical benefits come with it, but for such people, it's an extra reward. The situation can be similar to someone who writes a helpful book, even if they'd never make one red cent (like this one perhaps, hope not—ha!), why else would they even bother, right? Obviously something else provides incredible motivation, making it "worth it" or "priceless" for them, regardless.

So, if you do your best, but the other person flies right by you, or if you do not want to go out at all, yet see the other person out braving the inclement weather, regardless, don't assume.

As additional example, again based on running--some avid runners' reasons can go far deeper. Perhaps they want, need or have already, "run" away from something, literally. So, it can be doubly wonderful, both real and emotional at the very same time, like a play within a play. If they have not done it yet, they may be "practicing" or "rehearsing," and afterward, they may be blissfully re-enacting their escape! Also recall the "Runaway Bride" movie. Thus, many people may be "born to run" in more ways than one!

Yet, even if driven, one can "run but not hide" from everything. For instance, consider a male who knows that his father died at a young age, in his early fifties. Especially if his grandfather did, too, he may see that as a terrible fate that he would love to outlive or out ('wanna guess...) run. Such a person may be even more driven or die-hard, running very long marathons, etc. But, he might really only be running from a ghost—his own!

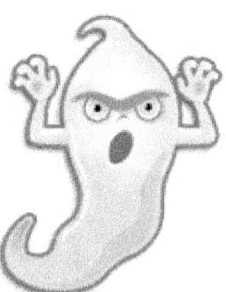

So, understanding how deep diet and exercise reasons can go can help you better understand other people, and yourself.

12. Gifts of Inspiration

Thus, the all-time BEST attitude to have towards others, regardless if you are taking their advice, trying to copy or be just like them, etc., is to treat them as INSPIRATION, guides for your own goals.

If anything does not work out, try again. No need to give up, get jealous, angry or frustrated, or try to get rid of their "reminders" of what you could be. Rather, see them as what YOU WILL be, once you figure out for yourself what works best for you. Why? Check this out: They are actually "there FOR you," perhaps even gifts given or sent by God, and you have free will to make the right, wise choice. So, appreciate them living ideals to strive for.

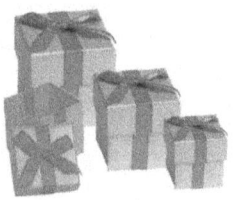

13. Fun for YOU

If there were just one secret about picking an exercise, it would be to choose what's FUN FOR YOU. "No pain, no gain," is NOT always true—there is a time and a place for stuff like that, but certainly not all the time. Most of the time, you should enjoy doing what you love and loving what you do. Then, when the going gets tough, like in bad weather, "your passion will pull you through."

14. Do What Comes Easy to You

Gee, here's a stellar idea: Why not start with whatever comes easy for YOU, then adjust or tweak it? If more of that won't cut it, add other things, but don't stop doing that, at least some of the time.

15. Days Off and Down Days

Every once in a while, we will all have down days. The weather might be adverse, we may not have time, be too tired, etc. But although a day or two off per week is actually BEFEFICIAL, and thus HIGHLY advised, anything more is a slippery slope, that can have a domino effect fast. It could be only too easy to get "into" something else that seems more fun right at the same time that you usually exercise, and opt for that instead. But, before you know it, it may be too difficult to get back into your groove. So, it's actually easier to keep doing things despite down days than let them go and have much more to do to get back in stride later.

To that extent, especially, remember: Less is more!

16. Changing Routines

If you are not starting out, rather in an exercise slump, change your routine in some way. It could just be temporary, or turn out even better than what you were doing before. Switching the time of day might be the ticket, or trying something new that uses different muscle groups, etc. A change of scenery can do you good, as well as getting away from everything for a while, a deserved total break. Afterward, you may change or come back, and enjoy it even more.

17. Stepping Up or Cutting Back

Some people might need to do more than just change, rather, step up to something more challenging or difficult. Yet, others might be better off cutting back, especially due to age or time constraints.

18. Not Everyone is Helpful

Always remember when you take other's advice, never to let them tell you what to do. Not everyone is helpful, with your best interest in mind. That is true even of your close relatives or best friends, who may have their own agendas. They may never tell you, but the truth can be quite different from what they do say, such as not wanting you to do or look better than them, etc.

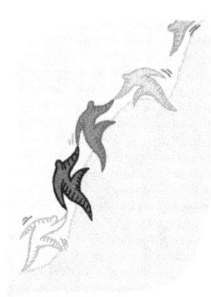

19. Gut/God/Grace

The best advice comes from you, yourself, via your "gut feeling." It is NOT merely emotional, rather very wise, so if you haven't "exercised" that, it's never too late to start.

Why? The truth is it's really God or grace, in silent disguise, so you must learn how to listen. Even if it takes a while, it's worth it, because although it's never fool proof, it's certainly far better than anything else. Once you do, you'll prove it to yourself.

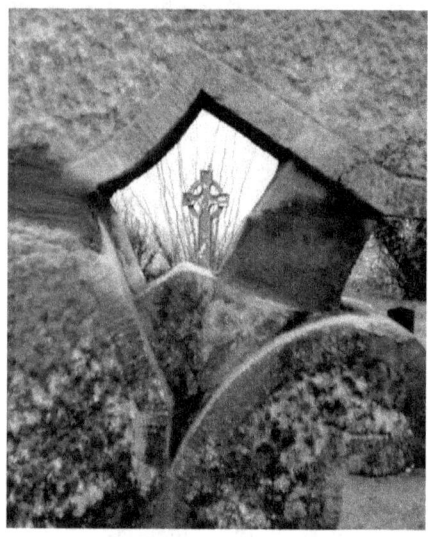

4
FINDING THE RIGHT FIT

A. Trial and Error and Process of Elimination

A very practical, common sense method of approaching many kinds of problems, not just diets and exercise, is "trial and error." It is a down-to-earth method that resembles a scientific experiment—the scientist or exercise/dieter has a particular result in mind, so they look at all the potential variables, try those that seem to work, and through a "process of elimination," get rid of those that don't to isolate the right one. But, what happens when your "naughty or nice" list doesn't pan out? What if nothing seems to ever work, after you think you have tried everything possible?

Answers include never giving up, and "thinking outside the box."

Obviously, never giving up means "going the distance" like Rocky Balboa in all his "Rocky" movies. Gee, did I just "date" myself, revealing my age? Yes, and I did it on purpose, to point out that those of us who are older may have to go a longer "distance" than younger folks. But, remember that younger isn't necessarily better.

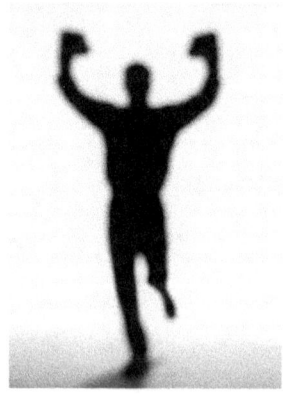

And, for those of you who don't think you are creative, here's a personal story that proves "thinking outside the box" is not hard. In fact, it might happen to you when you least expect it. Those of you who may need extra motivation, also know that it can occur like a wonderful surprise, even during a period of despair.

B. My Carb Answer Story

I've always been around the same weight. One reason is because it's easy to know what NOT to do, such as AVOID high calorie food lacking nutrition. Hardly any amount of beneficial exercise could reverse all the consequences. Yes, I had to fight my Italian parents tooth and nail---I was NOT letting them make me a prisoner within my own body, living under layers of fat, just because they thought it would more easily catch a husband or keep me warm in cold Pittsburgh! But, even later on, such as when I lived within my university's dorms, and I could eat what I wanted and run as much as I liked, I still never really knew what TO do.

So, notice the big difference between knowing what NOT to do, and what TO do. The answer can give you something far better than just correct diet and exercise, namely, peace of mind! Figuring it out is really worth it, because once such "paradise" is found, it can provide inner peace or the Peace of Christ, which is priceless!

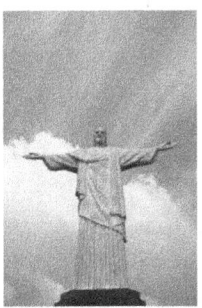

Believe it or not, I found mine during my terrible divorce, the very depths of despair, when I was suddenly back living with my parents! I woke up in hell all over again even though I had moved to warm, sunny Clearwater, Florida, where my job had been benevolently transferred. It was worse than ever, since I had so many new problems, including a social divorce "scar," by which, according to my Mom, I had "shamed" my whole family. You can just imagine the specifics. Does life get any worse than that?

Finding a job after it, however, was easy, so I found my solace one morning on my way to work when I noticed a new coffee and bagel bakery. I bought a bottomless mug and two sesame bagels, fully intending to eat one for breakfast with coffee, and save the other for lunch. You guessed it—the other one was gone right after the other. It happened so fast, it almost surprised me.

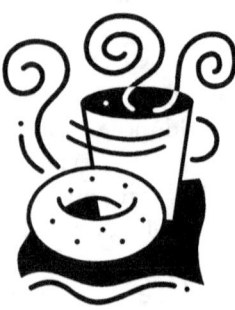

Luckily, by then it was time to start my 8-5 work day, so I had no time to worry if I had made a big mistake. Then, a miracle happened: That whole morning, I felt so good that I couldn't even believe it. And, I do mean the "whole" morning, because when lunch time arrived, I wasn't even hungry. So, I took my one-hour lunch at 1 p.m. instead of noon, and received another surprise— there were less people outside, so I enjoyed walking around more. But, I also accomplished a lot more work, so I could cruise through the afternoon, and slow down around 3 p.m., when I normally need a snack to get me through the last two hours, because I had all my work done! It also gave me many other choices as to what to even have for lunch, which also saved me money. I could go on and on, but you get the idea—this had an awesome domino effect that rippled through my whole life. So, at first I wondered if I should repeat it the next day. After I tried it again, there was no doubt in my mind that I had finally found my answer, because based on it, it was easy to figure out what to do the rest of the day.

Instead of bigger, fancy lunches, which I was never fond of, even if the company was buying, I brought a small sandwich, yes, with two slices of "carb" bread, and usually ham and cheese. That and a Diet Coke was all I needed. Then, for my 3 pm snack, I brought a some mini pretzels, which gave a "carb" kick to my mid-afternoon energy pick me up. Yet, the pretzel goal was to actually to fill a salt craving, which I always seemed to have at that particular time of day, instead of avoiding it. Later on, I also added another carb snack around 5 pm., right after leaving work, as if celebrating the exodus, and a fruit snack around 6, to tide me over until dinner. Of course, during dinner, I mainly ate OTHER food groups, for balance, and made a point to include a piece of fruit at the end, which seemed to work like a charm, the perfect ending.

Jovial note: To come up with the rest of that, I had to get rid of various stereotypical thinking, such as fruit is only eaten by old people—ok—REALLY old people!

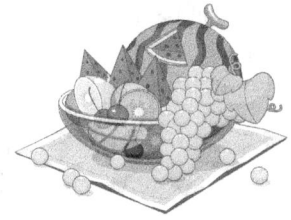

Yet, I really did have to get rid of limiting ideas things others had taught me, such as restricting salt. But, if you take a longer look at what I did, before you think it sounds too crazy notice this—it is really just a well-known, well-respected and well-utilized concept of "**carb loading**." I just did it **earlier** than most people, who typically carb-load during dinner before a race the next day, and I did it **regardless of any race**. But, it works for me because I am the type of person who's mind is racing, i.e. multi-tasking, even when I am just sitting, and those kinds of easily burned-off carbs can be easily eliminated just by thinking too much or worrying, etc. Since I do it when I think the most, it is like giving my mind a "bone to chew on" that both keeps it busy and energetically happy.

So, notice that although it began during hell, it was a "match made in heaven" that created heaven on earth!

C. Why No Falling Off the Wagon

Once you find something that makes you feel that good ALL DAY

LONG, you may never go back, and it is EASY not to "fall off the wagon," no matter what happens. In fact, you may never feel you are holding yourself back from anything, rather, basking in carb-heavenly joy! So, deviating would be silly or stupid, nothing you'd ever want to do.

I will underscore this again to eliminate another wrong assumption: People wrongly think that thin people hold myself back from eating what they want, whereas I already do! Duh!

Some also think it's strange to decline whatever stupid thing they offer, as if I somehow can't see the sinister look on their faces, as they assume it would be that easy to get me to fall off that wagon. Fat chance! I'm too smart for that. Guess what: Once you figure this out for yourselves, you will be, too.

D. Profound Peace

And, as if that were not enough, the peace of mind or inner peace that comes with it is certainly priceless, like the Peace of Christ.

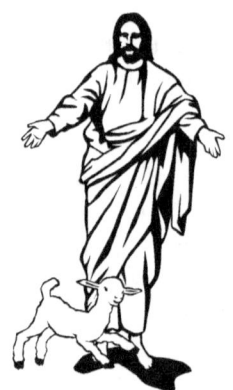

E. It Could Happen to You

So, the point of this whole story is to show you that going through difficult hoops to find it may NOT be the answer—it may happen TO you when you least expect it, even during dire circumstances, and it can be so good, you may never go back.

Yet, that is not the whole story. Its beginning occurred many years before, and since most of yours did, also well, let's look at the emotional underpinnings---the real reason it works so well!

F. Emotional Underpinnings

I had a terrible childhood, but there was a particular time when it became downright dismal, the "perfect" setting for an earlier miracle. Here's what happened:

When I was nine years old, we received news that my maternal grandfather in Italy was gravely ill, suggesting we should visit him before he died, as soon as possible! Instead, to save money like a mean, selfish miser, my Dad waited for months to book the trip. You guessed it: By the time we arrived, he was already dead, and when someone dies in Sicily, let alone the rest of Italy, everyone dresses in black and acts like they are walking dead, themselves, out of grief, of course. No one goes out, even to church (imagine that!), let alone does anything fun, but we were going to be stuck there for four whole weeks and I was only nine, so that long duration would have also been especially unfair to a young child.

So, one day, my Mom did something VERY uncharacteristic, that surprised me to no end—she let me take a walk, all by myself, wherever I wanted. Wow. Since I couldn't believe it, she quipped that just about everyone in the whole town was a friend or relative, so there was no need to worry. Suddenly having unfettered freedom with her blessing was wonderful, but I was in a foreign country, so I walked slowly and cautiously. Everywhere I went, people did indeed nod, smile and wave at me as if they knew me. So after a while, I felt more comfortable, and decided to hike up a hill, having no idea where it would lead. At the time, I was "following my feet," as they say, not really anything else.

But soon thereafter, I suddenly smelled something amazing, so I started following my nose, literally, with glee! I could tell it was bread baking, but I could not identify what else until I entered the bakery. I will never forget what I saw—bread baked in twists, with sesame seeds on top. It was love smelled at first sight! But, the best thing of all was that the baker smiled and GAVE me a free one immediately. That was the total opposite of how my parents always treated me, so you see, I received far more than just a free sesame bread twist, namely, the HOPE that my life would someday be very different, namely, just as FREE!

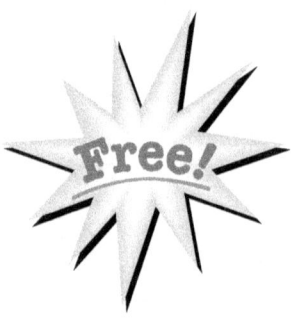

So, now you know all the emotional and psychological reasons (can you say FREEDOM?!?!) as to why I delight in seeing and smelling let alone eating, anything that reminds me of that miracle. The closest I ever found a very long time later here in America were, in fact, those sesame bagels. Thus, you also have to also add and account for the feeling of finding paradise lost. Once found, I truly found paradise, in so many ways, both inside and out.

G. Find Your OWN Paradise!

Although you are certainly welcome to, please do not take these two stories too literally. I do not expect the rest of the world to suddenly have two sesame bagels and coffee for breakfast every morning—even I don't always get to do that. Instead, go deeper than the specifics to the emotional and psychological levels.

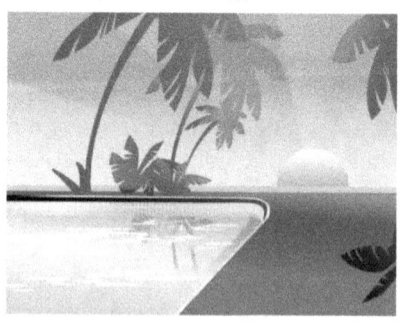

THAT is what you need to find, and each of you can only do that for yourselves. If a particular food item or type of exercise that YOU chose for yourself makes you that happy, then it is likely to have a beneficial, if not an amazing, far-reaching domino effect.

H. Address Cravings the Right Way

Moreover, take this advice with a grain of salt, adding things like salt, in fact, where and when YOU prefer. Avoiding cravings is a recipe for disaster. Instead, smartly include and enjoy them.

I. Make it More Special

Most importantly, feel free to add other things throughout the day that continues the feeling without adding calories, guilt, etc.

J. Drink More Water

Water is what your body wants most. Since it also cuts down potential food space, drink it with meals, but more importantly, drink it in between meals to keep hunger at bay.

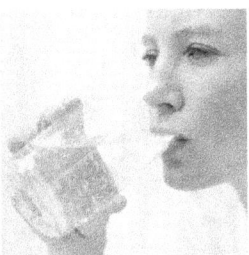

K. Tasty Tricks

Sorry to say, water can't always cut it. As good as it is for you, I couldn't imagine drinking it all day. If that works for you, then kudos, but if not, consider flavored water. You can make your own flavored water just by adding a little bit of juice, or a piece of fruit, such as from lemons, limes, oranges, etc.—you pick.

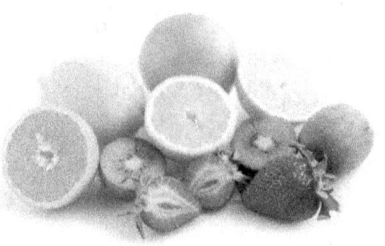

But, there will be times when you might need a tasty teaser, something to TRICK your body into thinking it is getting some real food, so other additives in flavored waters may be just the ticket. Same for diet drinks—their fizz may be worth the sugar substitutes. But, if you want to avoid certain substitutes, check labels because certain brands such as "SoBe" do use more natural options, like "Truvia." Again, pick and choose and try things out until you find what works well or best for YOU.

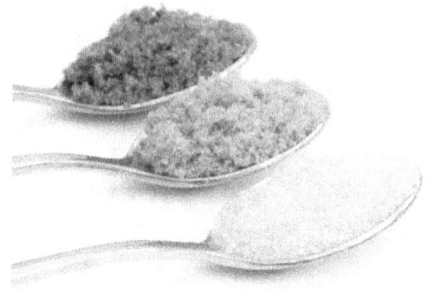

L. Diet Drinks

Even if you dislike Diet drinks, especially sodas, please understand that some of us love and prefer them, so we don't drink them to diet. Instead of sacrificing, we actually like them BETTER, whereas we may really dislike regular colas or juices. We are NOT settling, and nor should you!

Moreover, the reason why we like them better concerns our metabolism, or specific body types, so let's look at them, next.

The Almost All Carb Diet…

5
METABOLIC BODY TYPES

A. Small, Medium and Large?

People seem to have three basic body types, small, medium and large--right? But, can they really be so easily placed into their corollary categories, skinny, regular and fat? Is there more to that? The answer is both yes and no. Here's why:

B. Don't Judge a "Book" by Its Cover

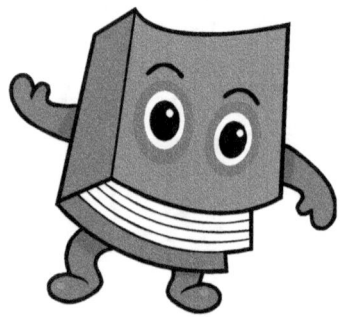

Yes, to some extent, the reason most people are thin is that they eat less, whereas others more, but that's only part of the problem. Another big factor is what they DO about it, which, as already discussed, is not quickly fixed by long, difficult workouts, rather, what ELSE do they do all day long? Yet, on the other hand, it would be just as wrong to assume laziness, because some really try very hard, but never seem to get any desired results. So, instead of judging mere appearances, or even those attitudes, let's look at something else, metabolism, which may be the biggest factor or all.

C. Ayurveda Advise

There is much more to the three body types than meets the eye. For a wonderful explanation as to how they match up with an ancient Indian, Hindu system known as "Ayurveda," please consult various books written by world-renowned author Depak Chopra.

One if his "diet" books has recently been featured on various PBS television channels. The reason why his stuff is so popular is because he, just as I do, too, goes beyond mere diet and exercise to address emotional and psychological factors.

Yet, he does much more than that. He addresses various medical issues both as a "Western" medical doctor, and by incorporating "Eastern" medicine, especially Ayurveda. He is also a very spiritual person, who has written many books on that, alone. The best way to address any particular issue really is to "treat the whole patient."

So, let's do that here, beginning with one more profound concept, a common denominator of all three body types: metabolism. Since a high metabolism is most desirable, yet has adverse effects, and can be very easily misunderstood, let's focus on that one, to understand it better and obtain invaluable insights about the others.

D. High Metabolism

1. Personal Passion

Certainly, people with higher metabolisms burn calories quicker, so they would fall into the small, thin or skinny category. But, that's not just physical. Looking deeper at emotional and psychological factors, one will most likely find that other things may be eating up the calories, as well, or even more than any physical exercise. They may be "Type A" personalities, driven by internal passion, fueled by emotions, which can burn off calories real quick. Finding the proper channel for such passion can be fun, but those who can't, or can't just yet, may get rid of even more as they struggle inside.

2.   Domino Effects

<u>Jovial note</u>: Some people can be so wound up internally (not just a Type A, but a double, or even a Triple AAA, like me) that a cup of coffee can actually calm them down! It can take them over "the edge" to inner peace! I remember when someone said that about me—they were so right, and we all had a good laugh.

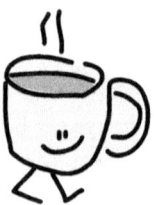

Yet, none of this is a laughing matter, because behind it can lie THE key or the answer! In fact, certain coffee (tea, etc.) blends can perfectly match a person's metabolism and work like magic. I have found two brands that work like a charm. They provide a domino effect, because they not only keep me happy, but stop me from drinking more of them the rest of the day. Some can even cure strange headaches! So, notice one thing can mean so much!

3.   Adverse Effects

Even a desirable high metabolism has adverse effects. It's like a double-edged or a "Midas touch" that can be great but have various consequences, so understanding it is very important.

Since calories are easily eliminated mostly by internal fury, such a person is likely to get cold too quick, especially in between meals. Others things that can happen include certain kinds of headaches, loss of concentration when blood sugar levels drop, etc. So, of course, one easy answer can be snacks intermittent of meals. But, cold may not be as easily fixed.

First, notice the irony that someone who may be so "hot under the collar" inside emotionally could even become cold so fast outside. Yet, the answer is usually NOT to "just wear a sweater."

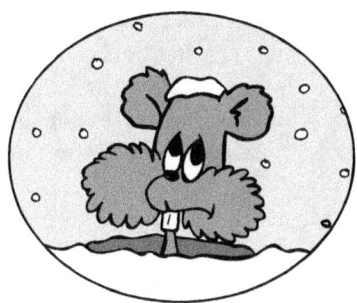

<u>Jovial note</u>: If I, who somehow survived living in cold Pittsburgh for almost 40 years, had a quarter, or even a nickel for all the times I've heard that silly "just wear a sweater" patronizing advice, I'd be so rich I wouldn't even have to bother to write this book—right? Good thing that's not my goal—eh?

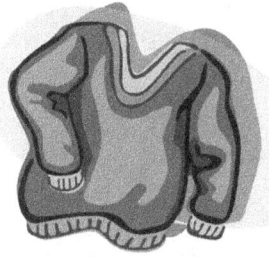

But, I mention that for many good reasons, including ones that concern the slower metabolisms of other body types. Get this: Just wearing a sweater wouldn't work for some of them, either!

A high metabolism burns off so many calories that wearing, say, five more sweaters wouldn't be enough! Why? Because that body type is also easily adversely affected by wind, which can also come in the form of air-conditioning. So, the tiniest area of exposed skin could make the rest of their body cold, despite six sweaters. Other people with different body types could sit by an open window, right under a fan or next to an air-conditioner and feel mighty fine, while others might not only be cold, but sneeze constantly and even catch terrible colds. Again, please realize that can happen just as easily to people with slower metabolisms and larger body types.

Thus, optimum diets and exercise go much deeper, to emotional and psychological levels, yet even the best can be adversely affected by other factors, such as improper climates. So, if a person notices after a long period of time that a climate change would be more beneficial to their whole life, they might have to make a big move.

Bottom line: Many things, big or small, can undermine or greatly enhance even the best diet or exercise. So, awareness is key. Instead of jumping to conclusions about body types or taking someone else's bad advice about wearing silly sweaters, each person must figure out what makes them tick. For diets and exercise to really work, a person must specifically understand what works and what does not FOR THEM, and do something about it. Sometimes, they will have to care enough about themselves, despite what others might say, to make a drastic yet wonderful change.

4.   Hidden Factors

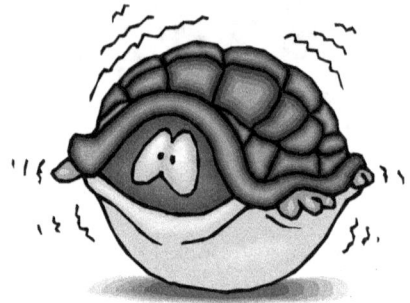

Although making big changes can be and fun, jumping the gun too soon can be regrettable. One truly must look before one leaps. Yet, certain things may remain hidden, regardless, so the best thing of all is to follow your gut/God/grace, for your own good, even if it means running against the wind. To get this point across, here's a personal example, prefaced with a poignant movie quote:

Jovial note: In a well-known movie, an oldie but a goody, called, "When Harry Met Sally," a comic romantic couple refusing to commit give each other both friendship and grief until the end. When Harry finally admits he loves Sally, he begins his long list of reasons with, "I love that you get cold when it is 71 degrees out."

That was funny to watch, because we've all "been there," having different, perhaps VERY different, reactions to temperatures than other people. Men and women can really disagree--usually one compromises for the other. For some, that's not a big deal, but for others, it can undermine their entire lives and well-being, which is NOT something that should be willingly compromised.

As for me, I was basically ALWAYS cold living in Pittsburgh. With the exception of a few summer months, which went by lightning-fast, I was cold when others were quite comfortable. Looking deeper, I was freezing from something else—all the caring I never got from my parents and later on, the terrible stereotype of female attorneys, evil things that rhyme with "itch." All my life I wanted to move to warm and sunny Florida, but everyone talked me out of it, deeming it silly and childish, but I never gave up.

In my early twenties, I obtained a job transfer to Clearwater, so I thought I was set for life, and when it did not, I went back to school, obtained higher degrees, and did more professional things. But, my inner child would not stop, so for spiritual reasons, after thinking about it for two whole years, five years ago I took a huge leap of faith and moved to the warmest spot of all, Key West. Now I am even more glad I did than the initial wonderful times, because now I am fulfilling my destiny by writing these books to help other people, because that IS heaven on earth, for me.

Yet, unbeknownst to even me, I was in for a quite a surprise. After sustaining two injuries in the same left sciatic area, and treating it is all sorts of ways until I figured out what was really wrong, I found out that my spine has been out of line, most likely since birth. In fact, I was born DEAD. My Mom has told me the story countless times, to make me feel bad for what she had to go through—right? See how cold? Both of us were so bad off because she had refused to go to the hospital until her water broke, taking an aunt's advice to seriously, so we were both about to die. She cared more about others, that they would laugh at her if she went to the hospital too early, to the extent of putting both of us in dire death jeopardy. A caesarian section got me out, but I was DOA, so they pronounced me and put me aside in the delivery room to prevent her from "joining" me. Within a few minutes, I came back to life, and started crying, so they leapt across the room to take care of me. I have heard that countless times from her, but no one ever mentioned any specific reason why. Something must have injured my spine.

Eventually, after trying just about every kind of Western medicine solution, especially various chiropractors, as well as many Eastern things like yoga, acupuncture, etc., it became clear to me that something else, far more profound, must be hindering my health. Once I understood that, I found my answer, and although I am never free of pain, I have not been back to the chiropractors since!

5.   THRIVING in Heat and Humidity!

So, the point to this story is that my desire to live in warm, sunny Florida was NOT CHILDISH! Here, I not only survive, but THRIVE in its heat in humidity, the more the better. That might not fit other people, but for me, it makes very practical, common sense. Obviously, a person who's spine has been stretched out of line since BIRTH could feel cold for even the slightest reason!

Most importantly, I say this because I have met others who feel the same, so if YOU do, too, know: 1) you're NOT alone; 2) nothing is wrong or strange about it, because even though it may seem rare; 3) it's actually a combination of very understandable factors.

In fact, I am finally quite comfortable here. I used to feel like a fish out of water, but here I found my water, my fit. As long as I stay out of long durations of high air-conditioning, I've noticed that I'm only uncomfortable heat and humidity-wise approximately 3 days out of the whole year, when it "wants to rain," but can't, during days I call "angry rain" which are similar to "ozone action" days up north. But, the truth is that we may have many more of those, so it's really me who is hot under the collar those days, internally fired up about something, which cranks up not just heat, but discomfort.

6.   Diagnose Yourself

So, all of this has been mentioned to provide a thorough example of what ELSE might be hindering or undermining, your diet, exercise, health or even your while life. It proves that in order to uncover, fully understand and appropriately treat hidden factors, one may have to diagnose oneself using only one's gut/God/grace.

Even if difficult, it will be worth the effort in the long run, because it's your life, and YOU are certainly WORTH IT!

7. However, Heaven!

However, if one shifts one's focus from themselves on to God, and puts Him, first, Heaven could be just around the corner! In time, or perhaps in no time at all, you could truly find paradise, inside and out. So, despite your level of belief, if any, read on, because the last chapter truly is a sweet treasure trove full of priceless gems.

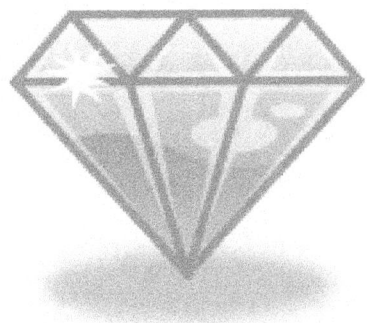

Guess what, your "worth" that, too!

But, before we do that, let's have some fun in the sun. Let's "bring it on," literally. Surprised? Don't be. Here's why:

Maryann Fenicato, Esq., Ph.D.

6
BRING ON THE SUN!

A. Darkness

Since lots of sage advice is already available on the deeper, DARKER psychological aspect of diet and exercise, this book will leave that be. If you readers want or need to "go there," please do. And more importantly, please feel free to compliment this book by researching and utilizing whatever other good advice, as well.

Instead, this book shall shine a meritorious light on something that could be VERY important, which may not immediately come to mind when a person is making decisions about diets and exercise.

Ready?

B. Sun Light

Sun.

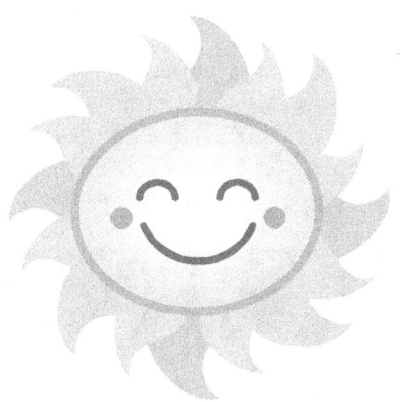

Fun.

Who knew?

You did.

Here's why:

When we were young, most of us loved to go outside in good weather to have fun in the sun. Oh, the joy of walking on a sunbeam! If that sounds like ethereal poetry, guess again, because all of us used to think that way as kids. We loved adventure, especially outside, and we believed in fantasy, fairytale things like ethereal magic that made life worth living.

<u>Jovial note</u>: If we found, say, a frog, we wondered if it would really turn into a handsome prince—hopefully without having to kiss it, right?

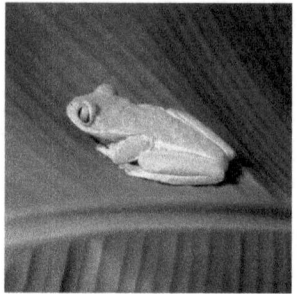

Seriously though, remember when just one thing, like an unusual tree with a huge trunk was like an entire enchanted forest to us? We were just pretending, or were we? Again, perhaps there was more to it than meets the eye, namely, we felt free to play, dream, imagine, discover, explore, and really LIVE!

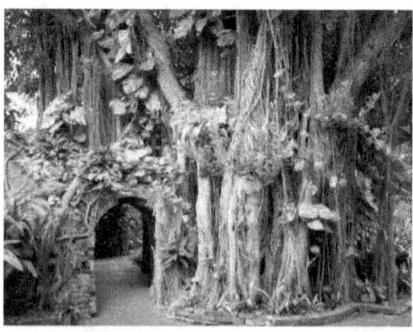

How many of us have lost that feeling?

What would it take to recapture it?

Wouldn't that be a great underpinning to diets and exercise, one that could pump all that up and escalate their benefits?

Not so silly or childish after all—see?

Get this: Jesus said we must be "like children" to enter the kingdom of heaven (Matthew 18:3). He meant we must believe and trust again, with the unfettered, exuberant, joyful hope, faith and love of a child.

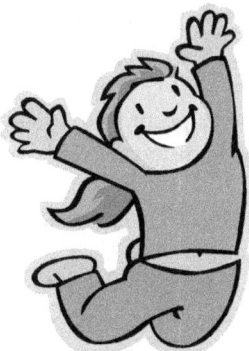

When was the last time you felt like that, especially concerning diets and exercise?

If you think they don't go together, guess again!

Remember all the stuff in the Bible about the garden of Eden? We were all supposed to live there! Duh! In fact, we did not sneak in, rather, God put us there. Double-duh!

Best of all, we can get there again in more ways than one, and even God wants us to return! Amazing--right?

So, before we discuss various ways to make diets, exercise and our lives more meaningful, in this chapter, let's focus on sunlight.

1. Magic

<u>Jovial note</u>: Paraphrasing the movie "Thor," the hero tells us that magic is what "science hasn't figured out yet." How about that!

Keep that in mind as we look at we think we know about sunlight.

2. Direct Exposure

So far, our science only has limited information on the sun, so instead of potential benevolent magic, the sun is given a bad "rap," potentially causing skin cancer, etc. There is certainly a lot of truth to that, so, although I love to bake in the sun, and my 100% Sicilian skin drinks it in so gratefully, I make sure to protect myself by wearing proper sunscreen and not stay out too long. I mention that because this section is NOT just about that kind of sun. Instead, I would like to point out that its emotional and psychological effects may be much more than science yet knows.

3. Seasonal Affective Disorder

Thus far, scientists have determined that some people suffer from Seasonal Affective Disorder, aka "SAD"—oh, how appropriate— right? This concerns INDIRECT exposure to the sun, namely, its light, which makes people much happier, not sad. The problem is that science treats it as a disorder. Here's why that's so wrong:

4. Daylight Savings Time

Gee, why would so many countries even bother to change their clocks and everything else that comes along with that, to extend and enjoy sunlight each summer during "Daylight Saving's Time?" Obviously, it's NOT silly, childish or SAD, rather, very worthwhile!

Duh!

So, why would people who need more than that be wrong? See?

Most importantly, however, let's take a deeper look, shall we?

5.   THE Son of God!

For many eons, people worshipped the sun as a god, such as the Egyptian sun god, Ra.   Later on, when many seemingly pagan things were Christianized, the sun's obvious power was still worshipped, instead as THE Son of God.

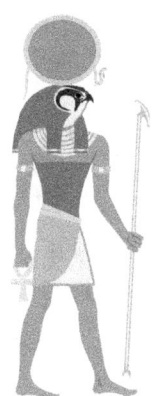 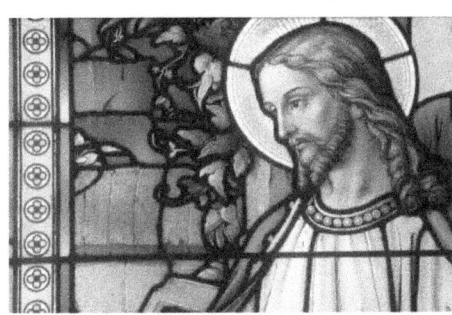

Moreover, many healthy practices, such as yoga, continue to include it, for example, as "sun salutations."

So, if a person suffers from "SAD" during the winter months when there is less sunlight, it may go deeper than mere psychology, and may NOT be a disorder. Rather, it can go as deep as one's soul, if is so, it is quite a different sort of problem, one that DESERVES to be addressed and to come out into the light of the sun, literally. If not, something that incredibly important, which may not mean as much to someone else, can ruin a person's whole life.

So, here's a story to hit that home:

6. A Mother Who Cared

I remember a wonderful, sweet lady who used to work with me. She impressed me because she was not religious, but spiritual, caring about others on a higher level. She used to tell me about her daughter, who became so sad when the sun lessened that she took her to shrinks, who of course, merely prescribed that didn't work, because they only treated the symptom, not the real cause.

Despite the "quick fix" failure pills, her daughter would undermine her life, by doing things like dressing unprofessionally when she went to job interviews. If asked later on, she'd cop an excuse, such as saying she was late and had no time to press the right clothes, but her mother knew better. Yet, luckily for her, her mother cared enough to see the truth, that is, WITHOUT blaming her or forcing her to adjust to the darkness. Instead, she did something amazing.

After I began working elsewhere, I found out that her mother had cared enough to find a job HERSELF first, in a much sunnier and warmer climate, so she could support her daughter, literally, both emotionally and financially, until she found a job, too, because she truly cared. Since I had the opposite, it warmed my heart, mind and soul to see a mother who cared that much and actually went as far as to change HERSELF to help. How about that?

7. Golden Light

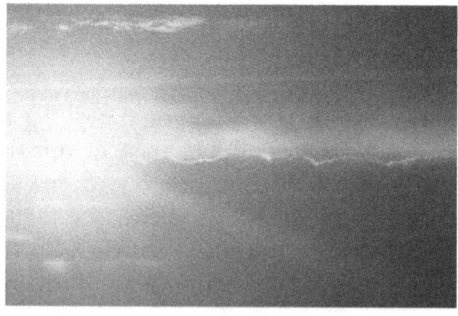

Yet, the point of that story goes even deeper.

It sheds a golden light on other things that could warm a heart, mind and soul enough to benefit a person's whole life or ruin it.

So, when you are deciding on a diet and exercise, look deeper inside yourself and notice if something much more important is driving you or crushing you. No diet or exercise in the world will work if you are fighting something on that level, inside yourself, because when you fight YOURSELF, yes, YOU lose, BIG!

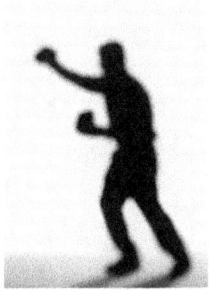

Yet, I will leave that to each of you to figure out on your own, because you are the best judge and jury of all—your own!

Instead, I will incorporate that story to move on to the most important point of all—how to make your diet, exercise and entire lives more meaningful, in other ways above and beyond sun.

But, for those of you who enjoyed that sunny story, know that it means even more to me. I took a huge leap of faith to move to Florida again, this time even farther away from dreary Pittsburgh, to America's Southernmost Point. I even include it in my exercise routine almost each morning, when I run to the pier and back.

Specifically, I bask in the sun, hanging out as I run in place to soak it up literally, but I also conduct a quick but effective, respectful "sun ceremony" right there, so that the sun and the Son "shines" on me the rest of the day. Yet, in so doing, I go deeper, all the way to the Golden light of God, asking it to splendor all my selfless spiritual endeavors, just like this one, done for each of you.

So, go for that gold—make your diet, exercise, and entire lives shine brighter and much more meaningful, too. Here's how:

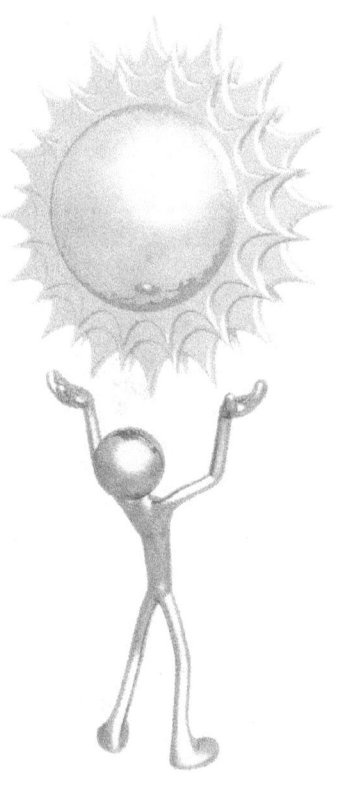

7
MAKE IT MORE MEANINGFUL!

The best ways to make your diets, exercise and whole lives more meaningful, and lastingly effective, perhaps even reaching the pure, enjoyable, easy bliss of nirvana (yes, that's POSSIBLE WITHOUT drugs, and I'll PROVE it to you), can be summarized, believe it or not, in two short, three-letter words: 1) fun; and 2) God.

Again, even if you are a disbeliever, do consider reading the last stuff, the best of course, about God, because I am not out to convert anyone. Rather, you might be surprised it its true worth.

But first, let's have some fun, literally!

A. Fun

In the last chapter, hopefully I had you feeling like a kid again, remembering your fun days in the sun. Ah, but who says they have to end? Your parents? Your friends? Your colleagues? Do any of them really have your best interests in mind, the most profound of all, going as far as your soul?

Notice again that Jesus, said we MUST become like children again to get into the kingdom of heaven, so why take anyone else's word above His? And, remember, we were SUPPOSED to ENJOY life, living in the garden of Eden, heaven ON earth.

So, why not have FUN while dieting and exercising. See?

1. Attitude and Perspective

Having such fun can be as easy as flipping a light switch. Here's why: You know what's fun for you. In fact, you know that all too well. Get this: The biggest reason most diets and exercise fail miserably is because they are treated as RESTRICTIONS FROM FUN, namely, what you'd rather do. And the biggest reason you do that, to your detriment, might be listening to other people. Why let them live your lives for you? Even those who do want to help you may be very different from you, so what they advise may not work for you. And, the prevailing trend is to assume "what's good for you" could never be fun. So, really all you have to do is change your attitude and perspective.

2. Freedom

You see, YOU hold the key, which is actually FREEDOM, specifically freedom of choice, aka "free will," yet another sweet gift from God. You can use it to open the "door" to fun, or lock yourself away in the opposite. Gee, which would work best? Duh!

Which will you choose?

3. Scientific Proof

Yes, ladies and gentleman, there is scientific PROOF as to why fun really works. Ready? Can you say, (drum roll, please...wait for it...) "endorphins" and "adrenaline?" Duh!

They are two specific examples of very potent and powerful "drugs," the fun ones, that is, with few, if any, side effects that your body produces naturally. Why else would a person get a "runner's high?" Now do you see how fun something natural like running really is? Why not fly high on that without regret? Yet, if it is not your cup of tea, no worries. You pick.

Pick fun.

Forget what others may say, and chose something far more important:

Choose YOU!

B. God

Now that you've seen that scientific facts prove fun is one answer, here's the better one: God. Best of all, I'll prove it to you without converting your disbelief, by showing you why you should believe in yourself. Yet, the best way really is to put God first, for yourself.

Here's why:

Jovial note: Remember the song lyric, "looking for love in all the wrong places?" Isn't it only too true?

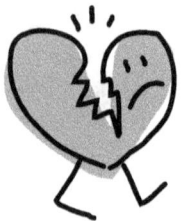

The same is true for diets and exercise, certainly a way of life. Let's take yoga as an easy example.

C. Yoga

There's a lot more to yoga than meets the eye. Some people have the wrong idea, thinking it is silly or impossible, only for people who can twist themselves into a pretzel.

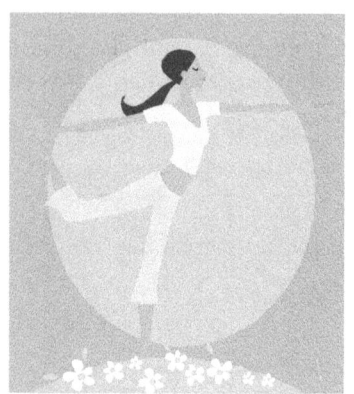 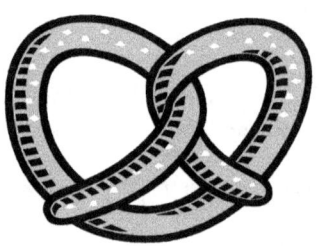

Jovial note: Wait, aren't pretzels on both of our advisable carb "hit" lists! This could take that to another level—right?

1. Simple, Not Difficult

I mention that for serious reasons, as well—some people skip yoga because they really think that's all it is—difficult stuff that few people can actually do. Now, I just happen to be able to do some of the most difficult, yet even I couldn't imagine doing other poses, so I can see it from both sides. But, those who can't see that yoga could also be very easy, that its simple stretches could be very beneficial, are really missing out. So, with an attitude adjustment, even disbelievers, of yoga's benefits, that is, could see the light. Instead of the wrong place to look, it could be one of the very best.

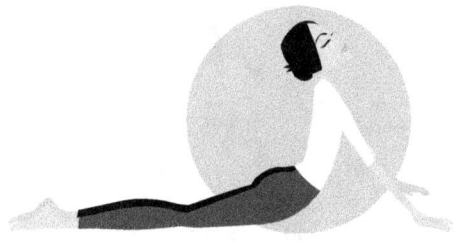

2. Going as Deep as God

Yet, the word, "yoga," itself, means "to yoke, join or unite with God." So, a person could use it to get much more than easy stretches or even a great workout. Instead of picking classes that omit prayers, one could put God first, simply by clearing one's mind of one's personal needs and problems. If that sounds like meditation, that's exactly right.

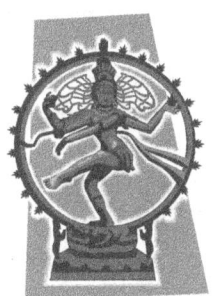

Yoga can be a wonderful moving meditation, a different kind of escape "drug," that takes you out to bliss. Thus, when focusing on something besides the pose, when one balances on God, literally, one can have it all, namely, both the physical benefits, as well as a yoga "high."

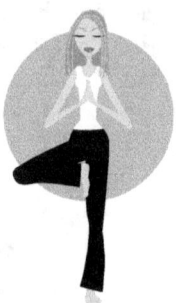

<u>Jovial note</u>: Best of all that high can turn pain into pure bliss. Why? Many times, when I am focused on God, not me, the pose or even just feeling better, my most painful spots can turn into God "goosebumps"---such a seemingly silly, childish or even spiritual term couldn't possibly substitute for boring, scientific "endorphin" PROOF—now could it?

So, check this out: Even non-believers could do something similar, get outside themselves by focusing on something else, and enjoy laughing all the way to the bliss "bank" on that, not God—get me?

D. True Bliss

You see, the error really is in looking for love in the wrong places.

Although others may have taught you that God is a mean old man, a geezer up in the sky watching your every move like a 1984 "Big Brother", or a bad Santa, keeping a list of people's sins to punish, to instill fear, the truth is the total opposite. Jesus told us God is love. He paid the ultimate price for that disclosure--his life.

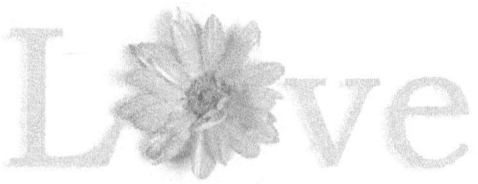

After that, many people, especially priests, severely edited the Bible, going as far as to selfishly omit entire Gospels, for their advantage. Instead of maternal magic, they wanted male patriarchs to rule, so they burned women as witches, held inquisitions, and did all sorts of other despicable things, purportedly in the name of God, to take power away from women and give it to men, abusing Christianity as their excuse, just like the Nazis used Nietzsche's stuff to kill the Jews. Here's the correlation: Jesus was one of those, too. See?

Guess what: Fire and Brimstone is quick discipline, an excuse or an easy way out for parents to control their kids. Many of them were taught that by their folks, so it has continued ever since. But, in so doing they may have purposefully or even just unwittingly ruined their kid's lives, teaching them the opposite of the truth.

The truth is God is everything benevolent, beauty, love, laughter, and certainly everything that makes life worth living, including childlike adventure, enchantment, wonder, joy, and certainly bliss.

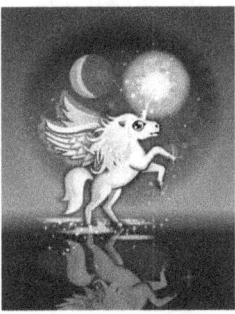

Jovial note: No, that's NOT crazy, I have lots of PROOF. Ha! I have done extensive research, some around the world, and every day, more and more of it is coming out, in books just like this. Ha!

So, see, Jesus can't really be killed, nor can love, because they both live in our hearts, minds and souls. And, those of us who are perhaps more courageous than others write books like these to get the truth to you, risking various things for your benefit.

And, most importantly, although meditation and nirvana can be quite easy, by simply focusing on what makes us happy, what's fun or blissful for each of us, the best way to make it last is altruism.

E. Altruism

Altruism is simply putting God first in your life, period. We have already seen proof that doing that can provide optimum results, perhaps even unforeseen blissful rewards for diets and exercise. Gong beyond that can be really astounding, truly amazing.

Again, each one of us must find the right way that works for us. Handing a homeless person money that might very well be used to buy alcohol might not be the answer. Donating it to people, churches or other places that are obviously not using it the right way, might not either. Writing books like this might be the ticket, or perhaps teaching a classroom full of students, but helping one person close to you within in your own lives could go even farther.

The possibilities are endless, most fulfilling when tailored to eachindividual, as personally chosen. So, I'll leave that up to each of you.

Instead, I'll end with an example of what NOT to do, summarizing this book's sage advice. It might even be entertaining...

F. End Example

As you probably guessed, here's another golden nugget, a story from my own life. Get ready to be astonished:

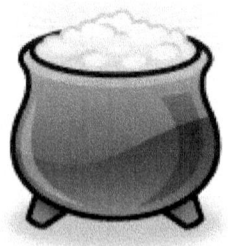

When I first moved to Key West, I had terrible neighbors. Most were noisy, but others were much worse. Two women in particular had it out for me because both of their husbands noticed me (apparently not them) when I went out running, especially. As you may also guess, there is much more to this story, but this will be purposefully limited to the running. Immediately, they got jealous and jumped to wrong conclusions, so they caused many more problems than will be mentioned here. But, what they did about running is just plain stupid and thus highly educational and quite entertaining, So, here goes:

The younger one used to run herself, but years ago, and certainly not during the early sunrise hours when I go. So, she was really angry that I "raised the bar" on her life, causing her, in her selfish opinion, that is, to have to go running, and at such an early time, things she thought she could avoid if I simply lived elsewhere. Yeah, right! Notice the potential disaster of such an attitude.

For strength in numbers, but really just as an excuse to give me dirty looks, she got a friend to run with her, who was obviously a more avid a runner than I. She thought that would put me off, but we true runners respect each other, so that did not work. Nor did the knee brace she put on as an excuse to avoid having to keep up with her friend—that just made her look mad, SAD and sappy!

She did not realize other people were watching, who easily saw through her stupidity. Many of them already knew the truth, so they would joke with me, saying things like, "who would even want her husband—quite a catch," since he looks exactly like the beer can he places on his Christmas decorations! His beer belly is quite large, like the rest of him, so his whole figure is not an hourglass, but rather just like a huge beer can, matching his block head!

But, the serious lesson here is that, by doing all those stupid things for the wrong reasons, besides ridicule, it also undermined the rest of her life, especially her work. She was too tired to do that, which, in turn, of course, just made her even more mad at me and herself. See how circular a bad domino effect can be!

Yet, there's more:

Although I moved, I still see her run. At least she now does it later on in the day, but I can tell that she's still very angry, thinking she has to do that because of me. I am not even there anymore, yet this continues. When will she let go the anger? Despite the running, how healthy is that? She still looks the same physically—is that really any surprise? Will she ever learn?

Ah, but now I'll tell you about the other lady. She was even more jealous because she's a lot older and angry at herself, although she'll never admit it, for not doing much with her life. She claims she's a business woman, but it's really her husband's business, and she's nothing but a 'wanna be parasite. As a result, she despises "young hot shots" who have done great things, so she is a neighborhood gossip, the kind that's always watching others, peeping behind her curtains. She has a nice garden, but her true personality is like the witch in Hansel and Gretel---beware.

Karma already kicked her once—someone stole all her orchids, so she's really stewing with displaced anger, not knowing who to blame. Gee, is that another disaster recipe?

Her husband was hospitalized right after I left, and people knew it was another karma kick, but she still did not learn.

'Wanna guess the end of this story?

Recently, I saw her, after all this time, and it hurt my eyes. Why? She somehow lost weight from doing something else, certainly not running, yet wears silly "short-shorts" at her advanced age!

But, that was not the worst part. Yes, she looks thinner, but too thin, and her white hair makes her look like a hideous ghost. In fact, she looks like the bad guy in the first Indiana Jones movie, "Raiders of the Lost Ark." When he greedily opened the glittering golden Ark of the Covenant, seeking selfish material wealth, he released something dark that shriveled him up, making him look like death with white hair, right before he turned to dust. That's exactly what she looks like, right before the dust. Will she ever learn, either?

The reason I still shake my head is that when she sees my former landlord, who's happily married, she prances around, as if she could have any chance. Fat chance! And shame on her, at her age! I bet her husband doesn't know—wonder what he'd do if he knew!

That's the real reason why both women had a problem with me—they were doing many silly, stupid and bad things THEMSELVES.

Obviously, both of them are backfiring, wasting their own lives, only getting worse. Even if they never learn, you can from this.

G. Farewell for Now

So, I hope you have enjoyed this book, and all of its facets.

Obviously, carbs, diet and exercise were only the tip of the iceberg.

Feel free to use all these carb-a-licious tips, jovial notes, entertaining stories, and sage, spiritual advice to your carb-vantage, but also endeavor to go deeper. Be a miner looking for true gold in all the right places, God and yourself, because ... you're "worth it!"

Jovial note: Since I already have and will most likely write many more books, perhaps even one focused entirely on what it's really like to live in Key West, for "educational" purposes, of course, (which will certainly be even more entertaining—eh?), here's wishing you the best.

So, instead of "good-bye," I say to you "farewell, for now."

H. Be Free!

Most importantly, however, above and beyond all the other stuff, remember that "what" ails you, may be "who" ails you, and that who, could be YOU! So, free yourselves--even from yourselves, and enjoy it! I dare you. Instead of just "bringing on" the sun, bring out the real you, and let it shine like the sun.

Bottom line: **Be Free!**

Note: In the event that any of you find any errors, type-o's, etc. please receive this author's sincerest apologies. We are all human, and "to err is human, but to forgive Divine." Far better to move on to write more altruistic books, helping others, instead.

ABOUT THE AUTHOR

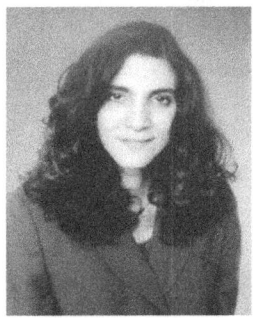

Maryann Fenicato, Ph.D., Esq., was born in Pittsburgh, PA, USA. From highly-accredited Duquesne University, she earned 2 separate doctorates in Law and Philosophy (Ethics), and 3 other degrees.

Currently: She's a "carb-a-holic," avid runner, a fun, charismatic, motivational, inspirational and educational speaker, teacher, guru, mentor and life coach, who travels domestically and abroad to speak in front of large groups at universities, colleges and other educational institutions, churches, youth facilities and other spiritual organizations, businesses and corporations. Yet, she also enjoys privately counselling individuals confidentially, especially troubled teens or adults who have yet to maximize their destined potential, inspiring God-centered lives beyond diets and exercise. A prolific author who's already accomplished an amazingly multi-faceted destiny, living the life she's always dreamed of in beautiful Key West, she enjoys sharing and showing others how to do it, too. For any such engagements, contact: mafenicato@hotmail.com See also her website: **http://maryannfenicato.com**

Prior Careers and Publications: She was an in-house corporate litigation paralegal for approx. 10 years, and a peaceful contract lawyer for another 10, yet winning any case or court proceeding conducted in Pittsburgh or Key West. Her legal and philosophical publication titles, alone, form a book much, much bigger than this! As also a University Professor, after teaching many things in many places, and winning 2 "Outstanding Professor of the Year" awards at PITT, she retired both careers "until further notice" and took a huge leap of faith, freed herself and followed her own true destiny!